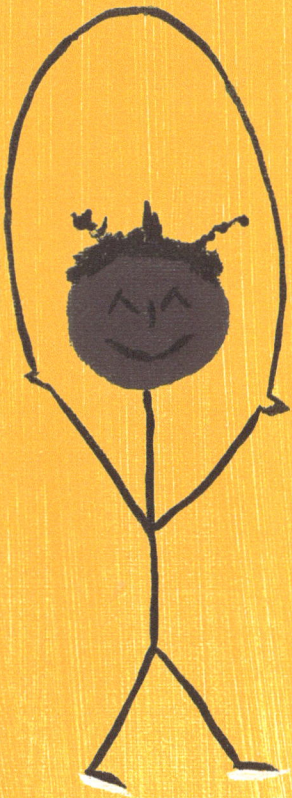

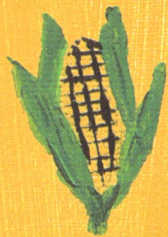

Corn

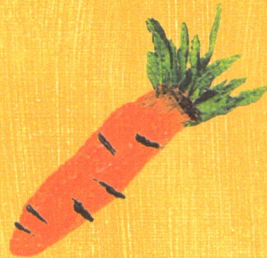

Carrot

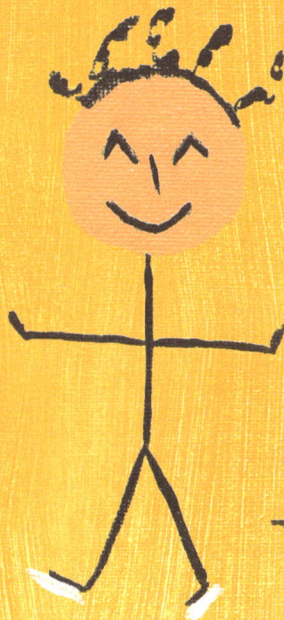

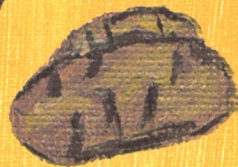

Potato

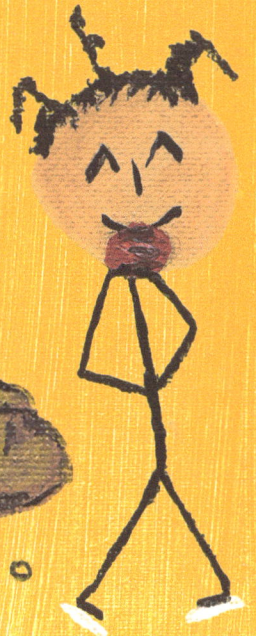

Let's Get Healthy!

ABOUT THE AUTHOR

Atta Van has a Masters in Applied Psychology. She has two children and four grandchildren. She believes the practice of healthy eating and exercise must be taught at a young age.

First Publication Date: July 2021
Revised and Republished: February 2022

Written by: Atta Van
Copyright® 2020 by Atta Van

Illustrations by: Zequeatta Jaques
All Art and Logo copyright® 2020 by All Around Publishing, Inc.

ISBN: 978-1-7344314-6-9

Published by All Around Publishing, Inc.
www.allaroundpublishinginc.com

This Book Belongs To:

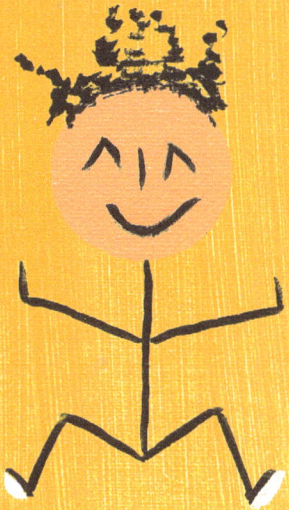

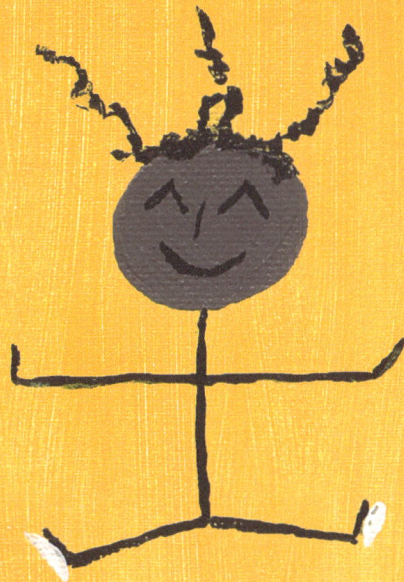

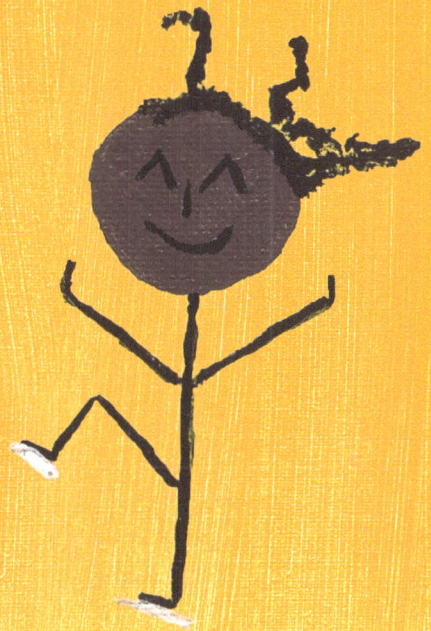

_____

Grapes

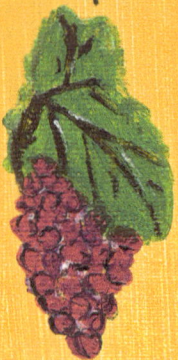

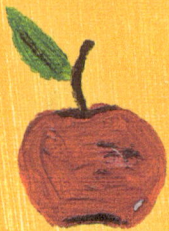

Apple

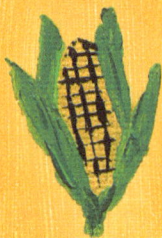

Corn

Carrot

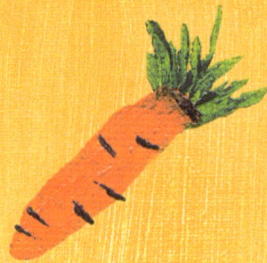

Potato

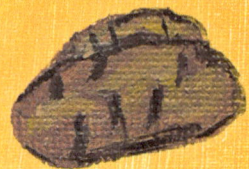

Pear

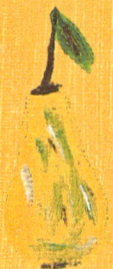

Let's Get Healthy!

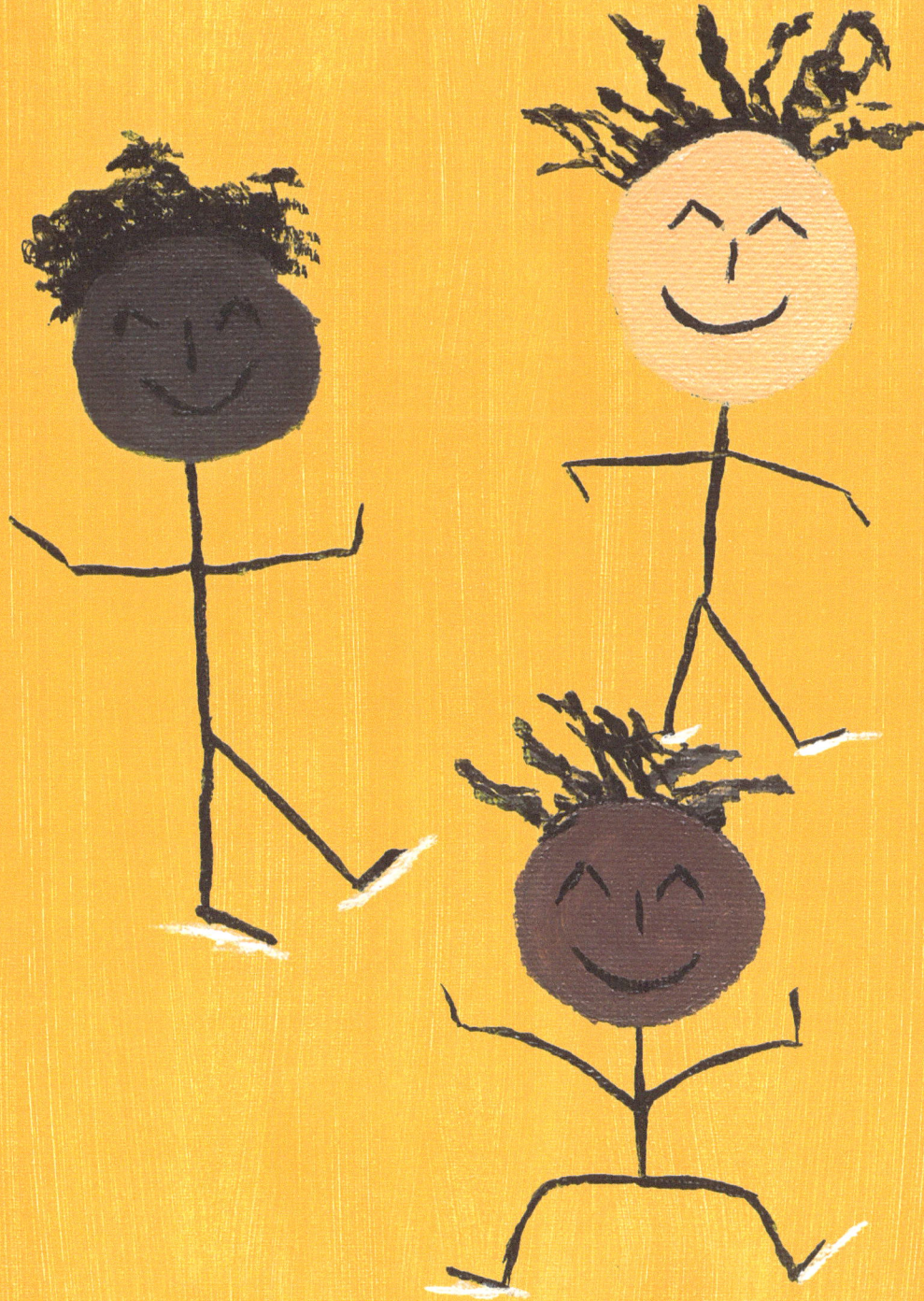

Written by Atta Van
Illustrated by Zequeatta Jaques
Published by All Around Publishing, Inc.

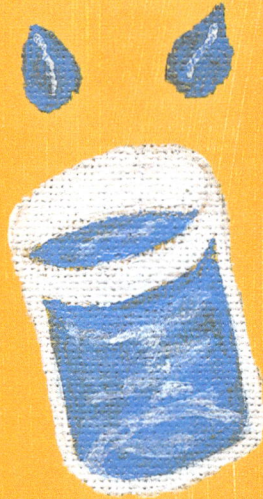

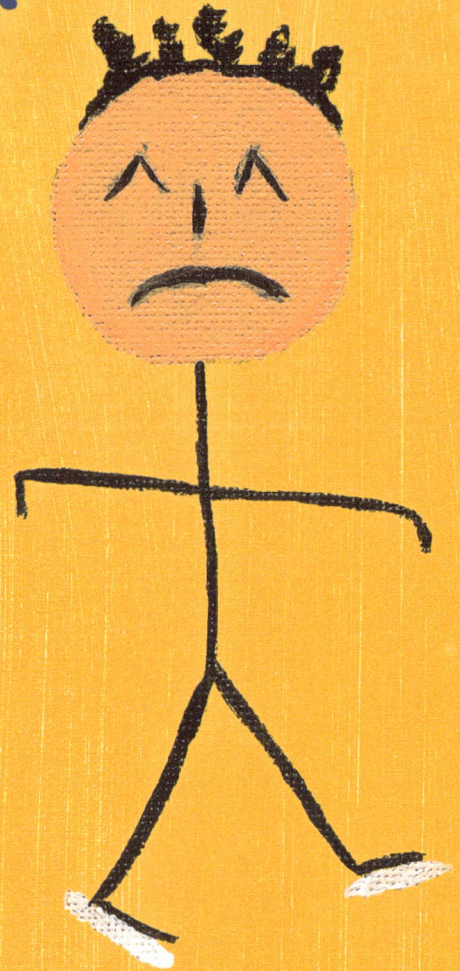

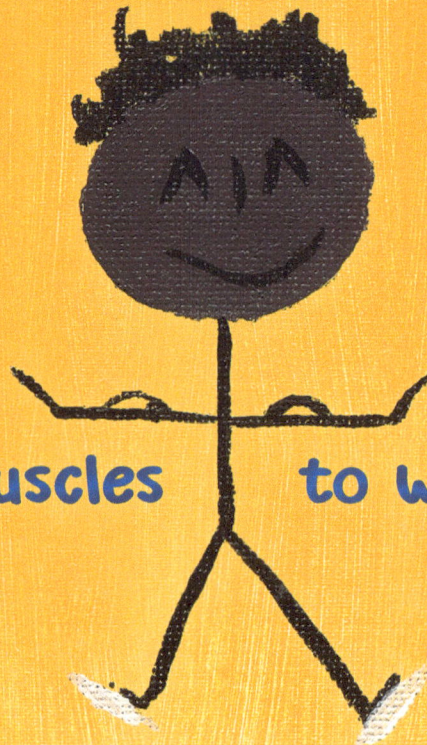

I LOVE WATER!
Yes, Yes, I do.

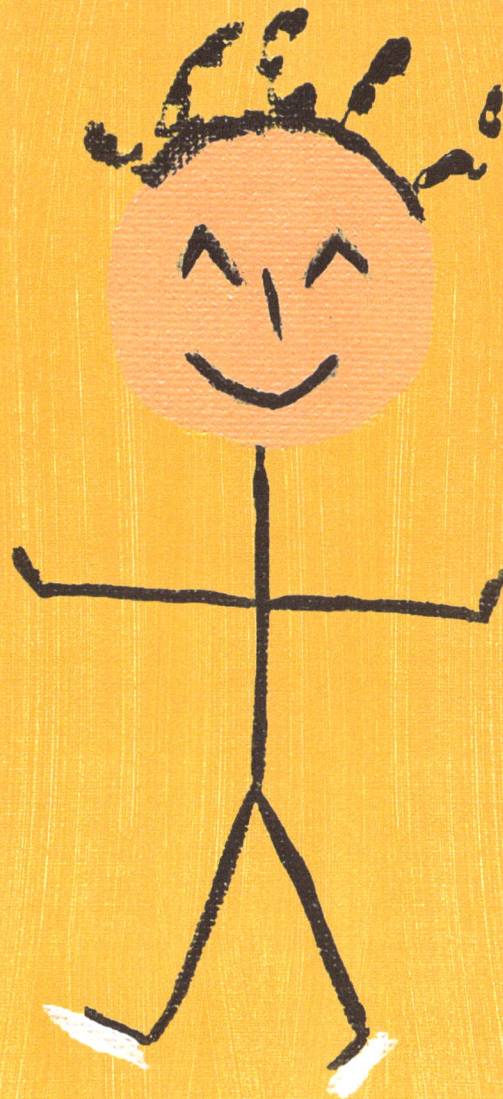

FRUIT
Why do I need to eat this fruit?

Fruit helps me to be smart.
Fruit helps me to grow.
Fruit makes me happy!

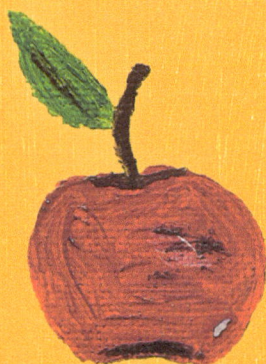

Apple

Pear

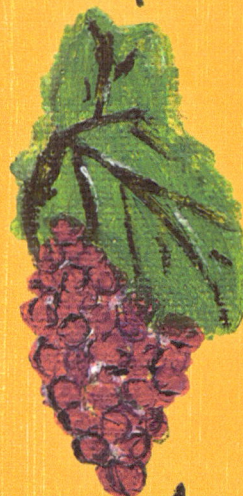

Grapes

I don't drink it.

No, No, I eat it.

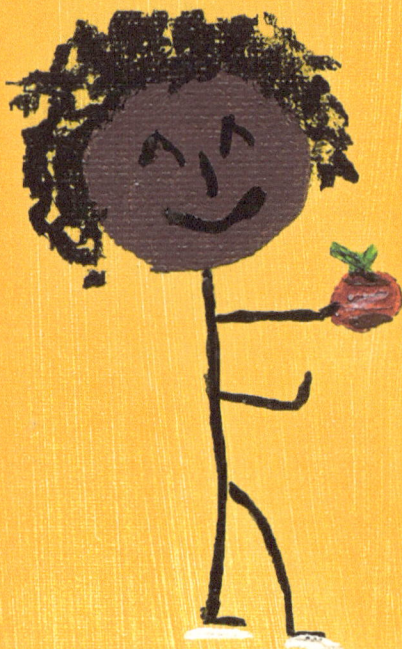

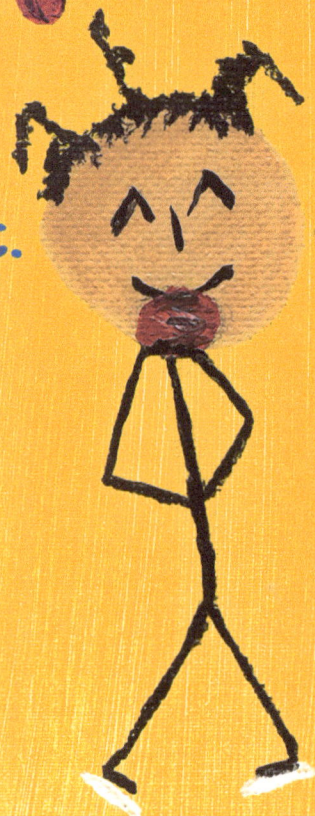

I LOVE FRUIT!
Yes, Yes, I do.

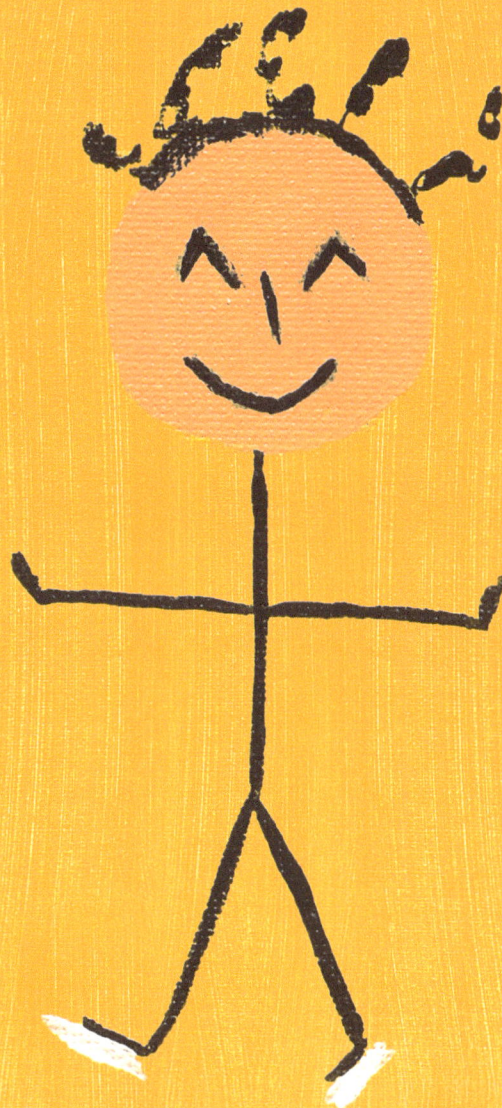

MILK

Why do I have to
drink this milk?

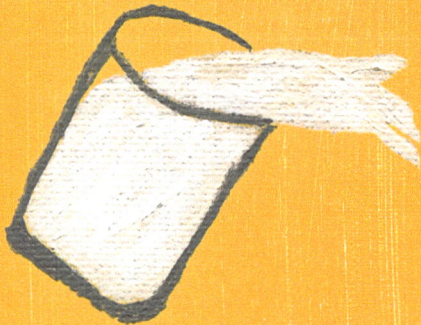

Milk helps me
to have energy.

Milk helps me
to grow.

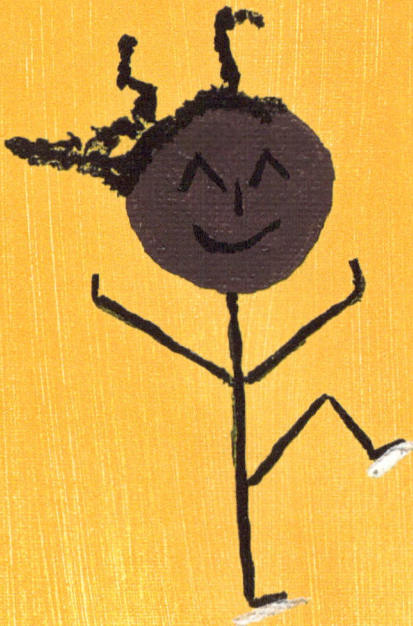

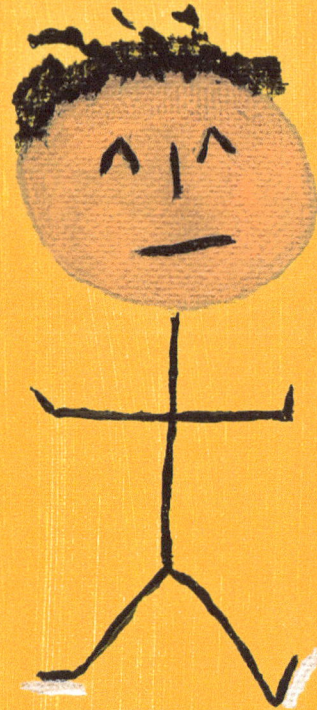

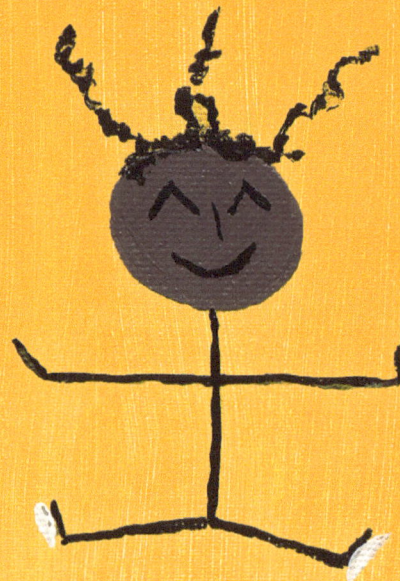

Milk helps my bones
to be strong!

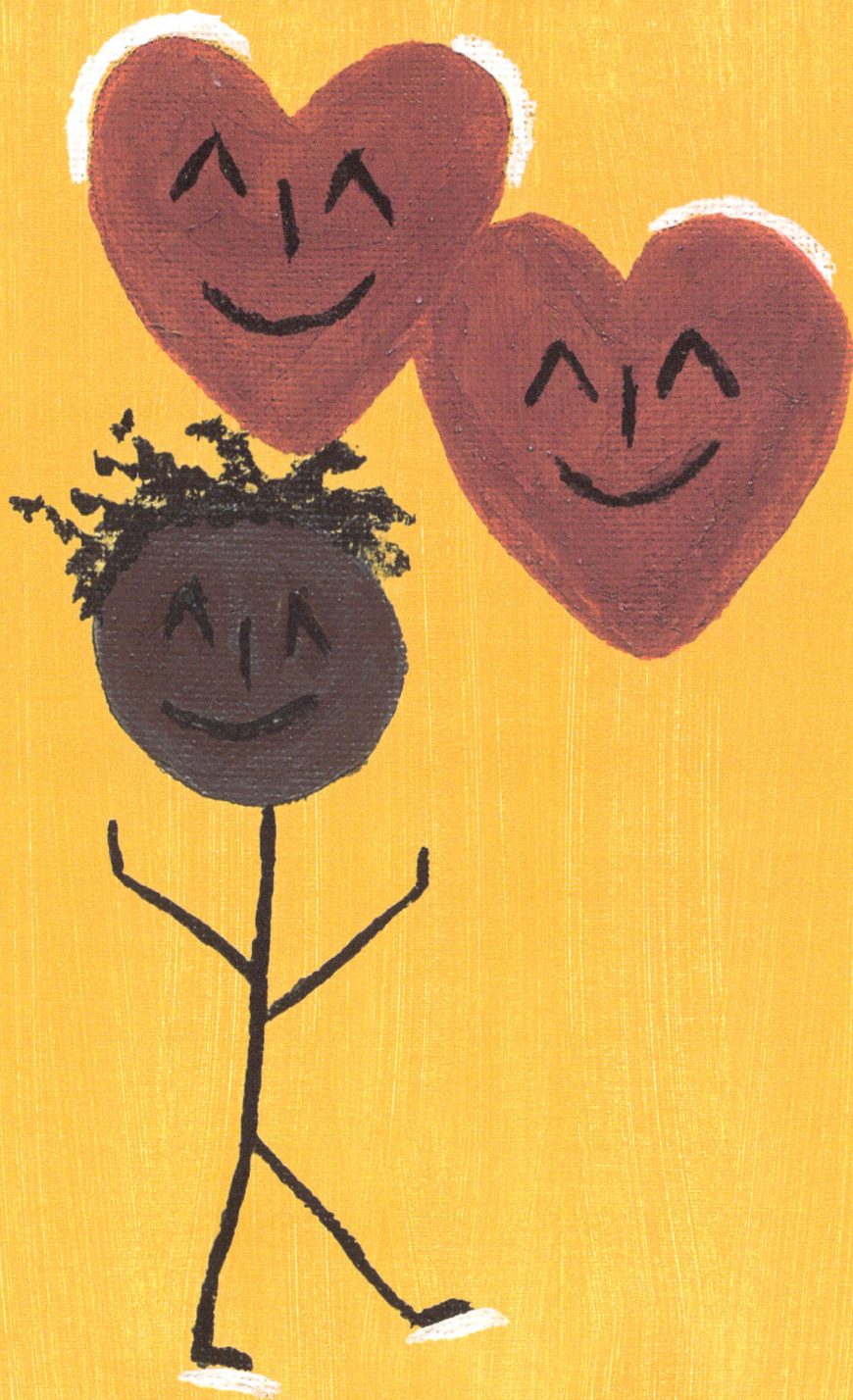

VEGETABLES

Why do I need to eat those vegetables?

Vegetables help me to have healthy and glowing skin.

Vegetables help me to have pretty gums and teeth.

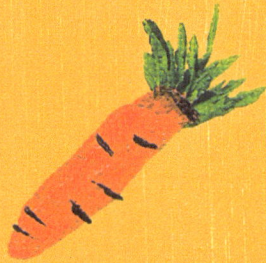

Carrot

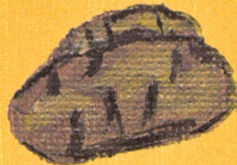

Potato

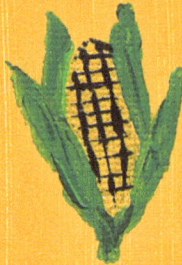

Corn

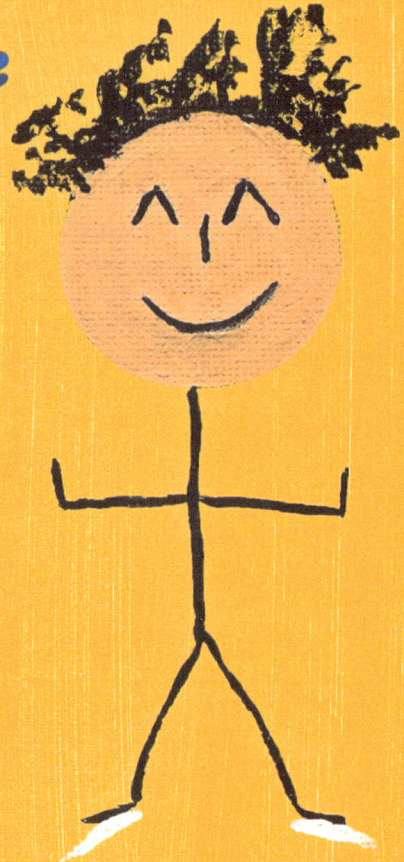

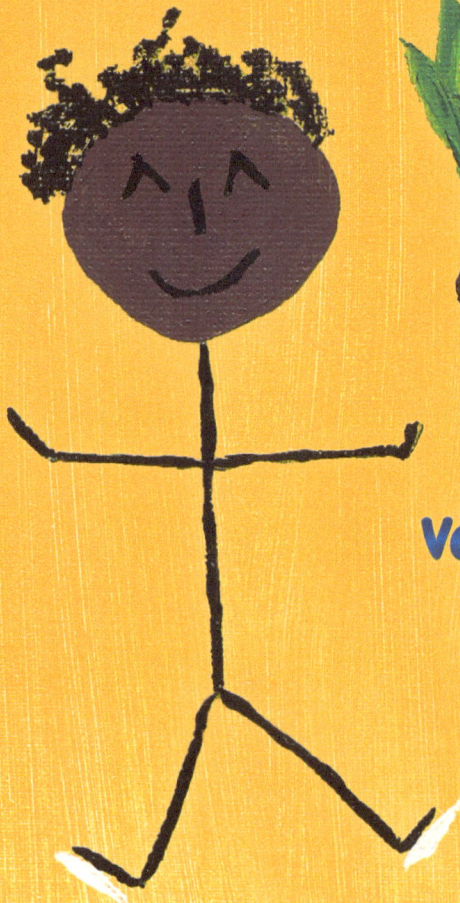

Vegetables help me to stay healthy!

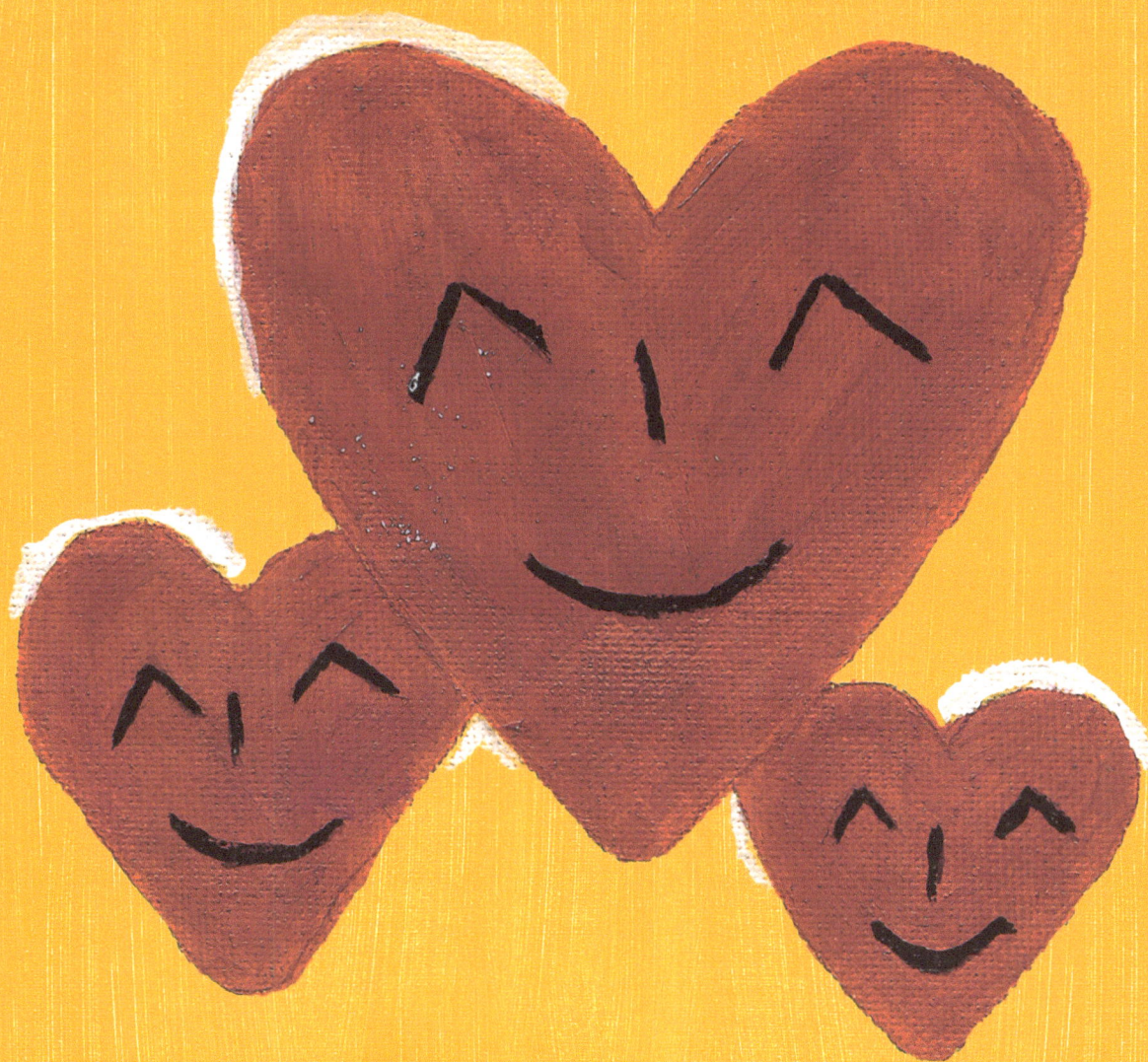

EXERCISE

Why do I need to exercise?

Exercise helps me to have a healthy heart!

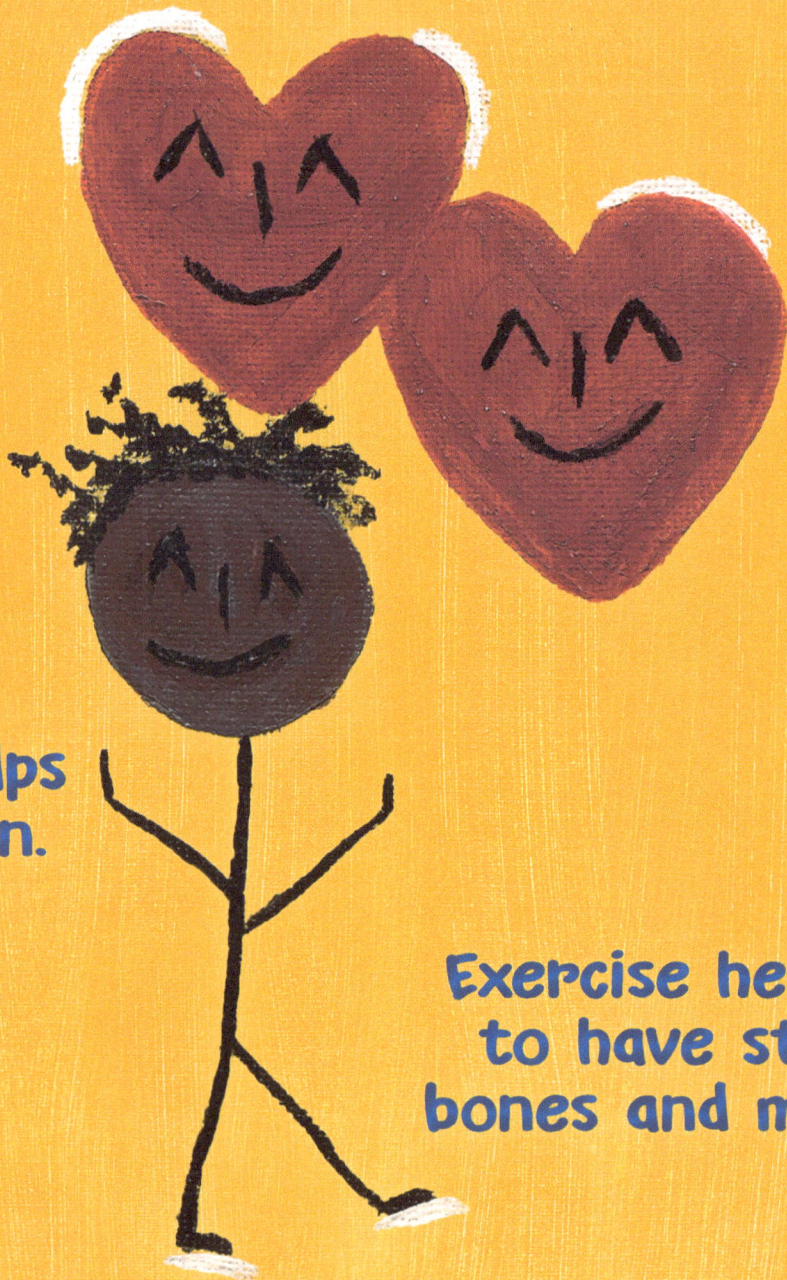

Exercise helps me to learn.

Exercise helps me to have strong bones and muscles.

Exercise helps me to be in a good mood!

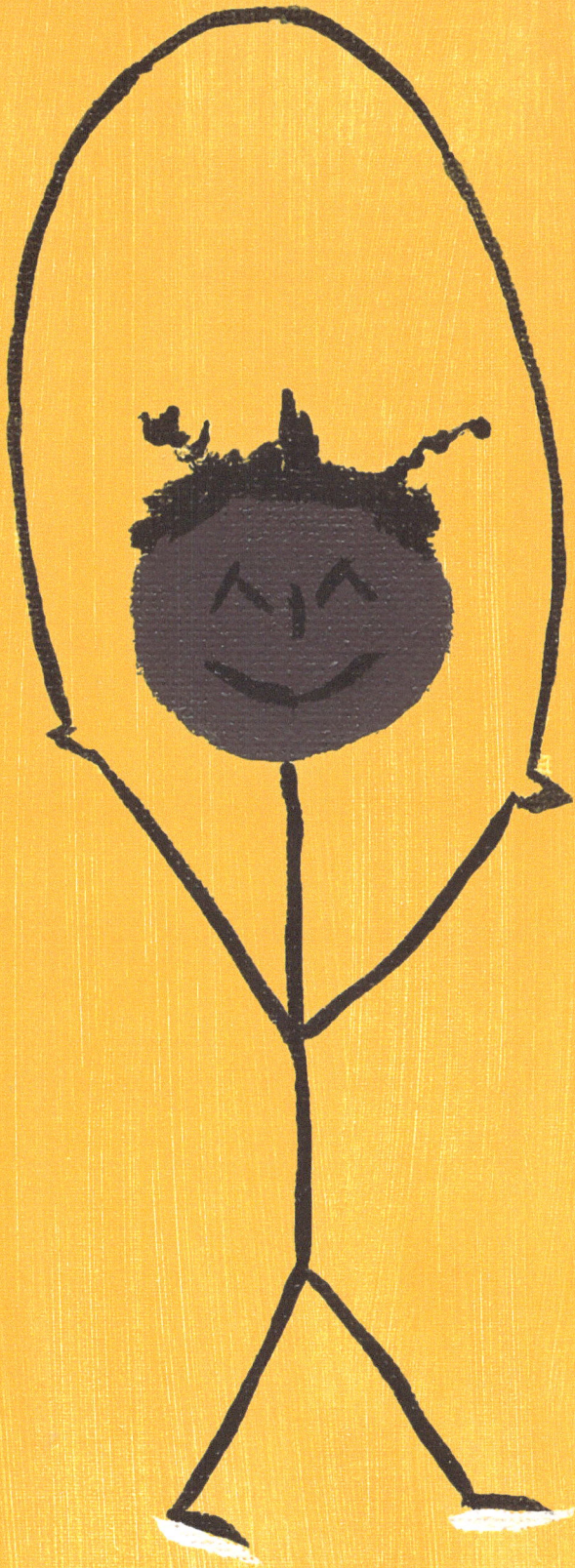

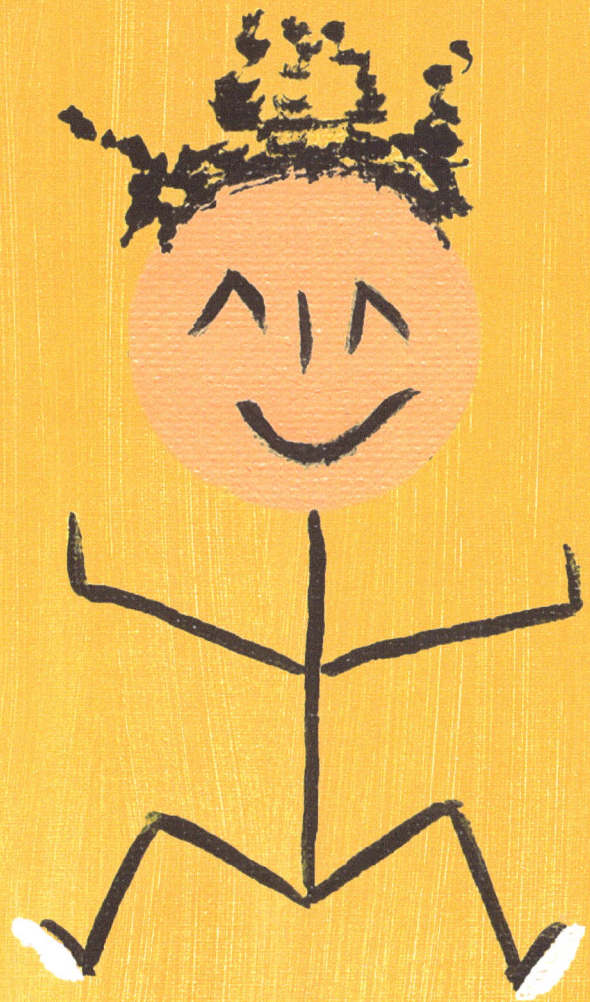

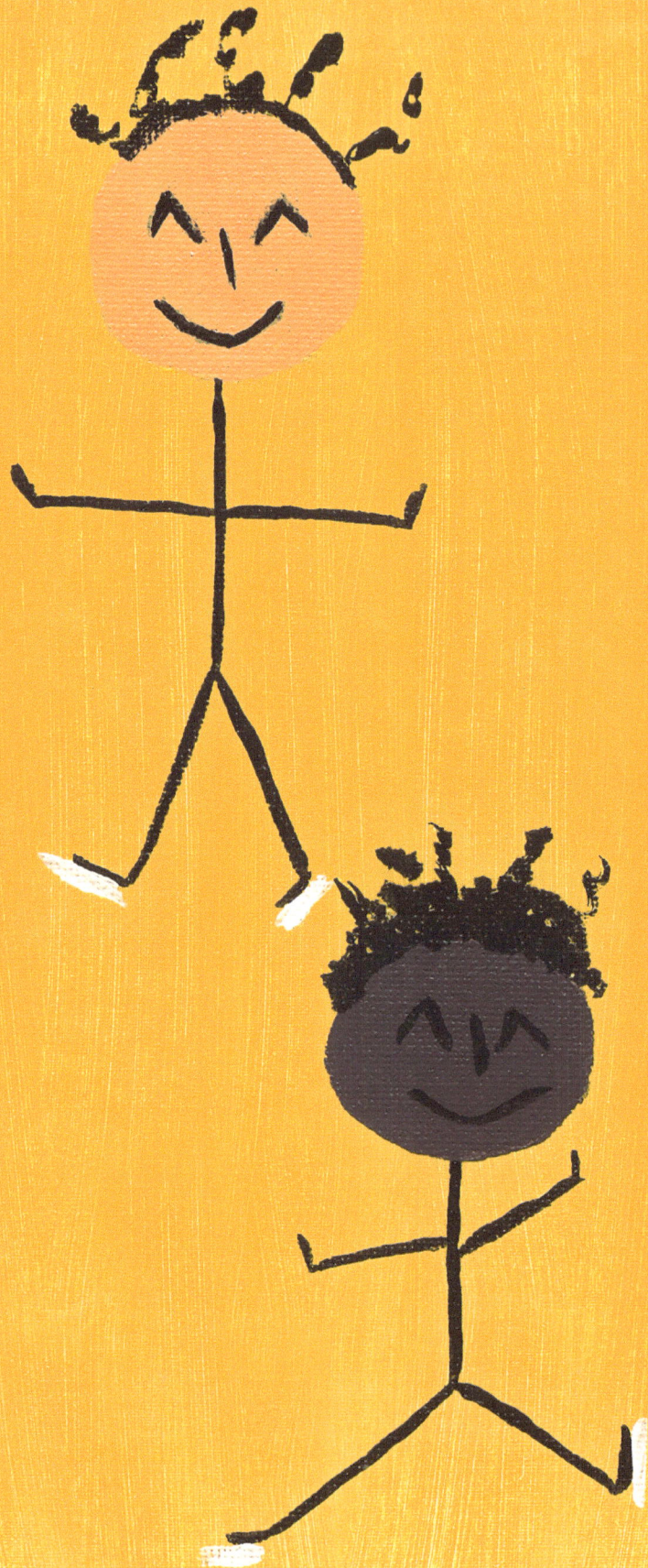

LET'S GET HEALTHY!

WHAT IS MY FAVORITE VEGETABLE?

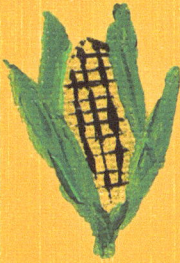

Corn

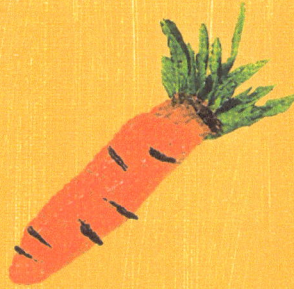

Carrot

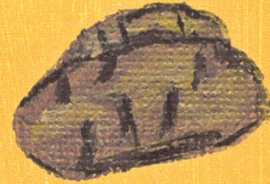

Potato

Write your favorite vegetable here

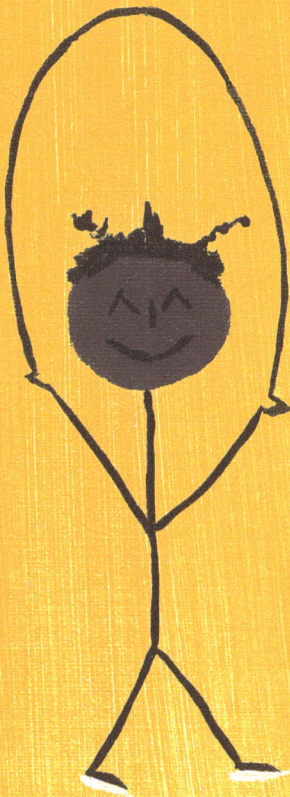

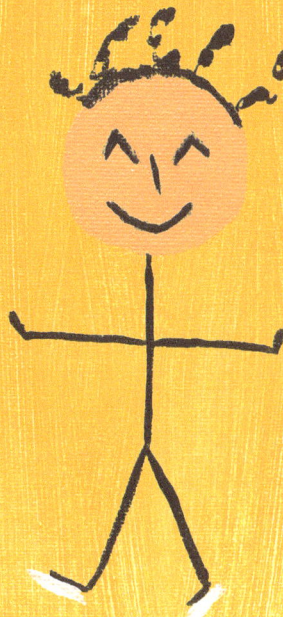

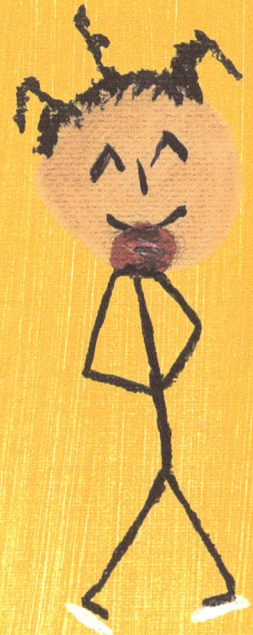

WHAT IS MY FAVORITE FRUIT?

Pear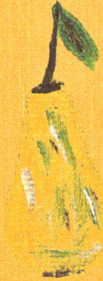

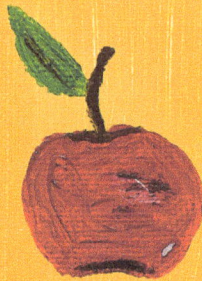
Apple

Grapes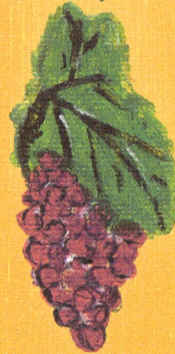

Write your favorite fruit here

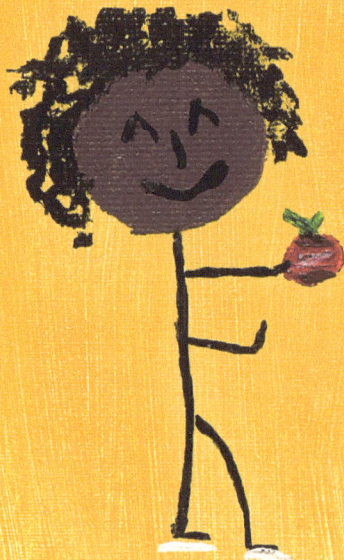 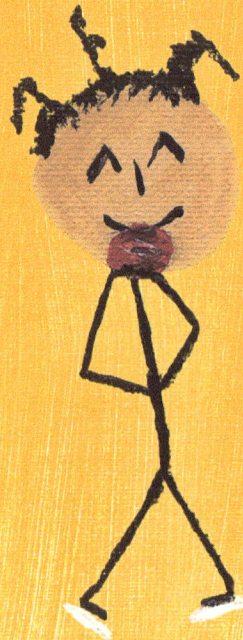

WHY SHOULD I EXERCISE?

Color in the correct box

It helps me to have a healthy heart......................................☐

It makes me sad...☐

It helps me to learn...☐

It helps me to have strong bones and muscles.................☐

It helps me have weak muscles..☐

It helps me to be in a good mood......................................☐

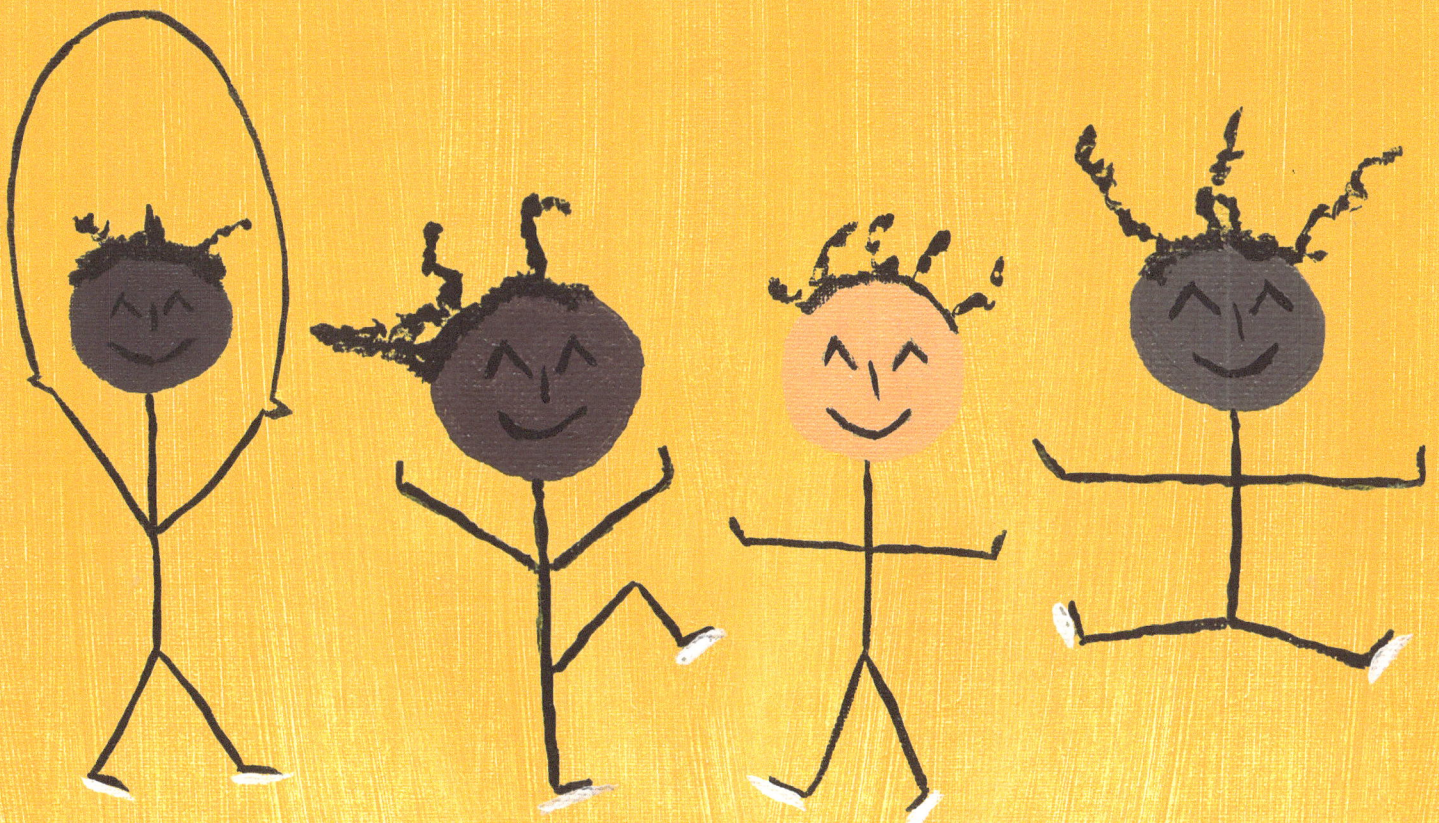

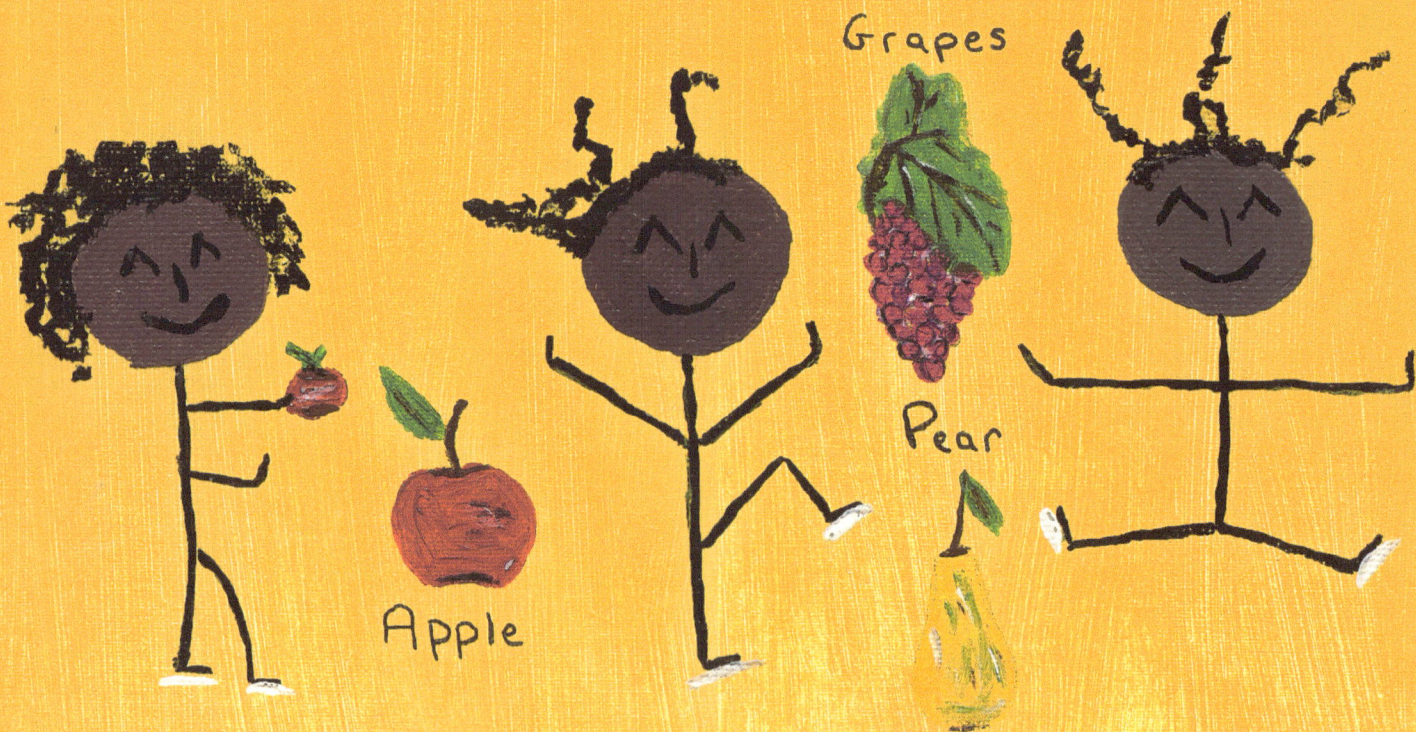

www.ingramcontent.com/pod-product-compliance
Lightning Source LLC
Chambersburg PA
CBHW061154030426
42336CB00002B/41